GUIDE SIX:
BUILD YOUR ROUTINE

*From Root to Tip: A Growing Hands
Guide for Natural Hair*

BY CONSTANCE HUNTER

For permissions, inquiries, or additional resources, please contact:

Pre'Vail Natural Hair Salon

www.prevailyournatural.com | prevailyournatural@gmail.com

This book is intended for informational and educational purposes only and should serve as a general guide to understanding and improving natural hair health. While the methods and recommendations provided are based on expertise in natural hair care and trichology, they are not intended to replace professional medical or dermatological advice.

If you are experiencing severe scalp conditions, excessive hair loss, or other persistent issues, it is strongly recommended that you consult a licensed dermatologist or a professional cosmetologist specializing in scalp and hair health. A trained professional can assess underlying causes and provide personalized treatment plans tailored to your specific needs.

By using the information in this book, the reader acknowledges that the author and publisher are not responsible for individual outcomes. Readers should exercise their own discretion when applying the suggested practices.

First Edition: 2025

ISBN:

Paperback: 978-1-968134-06-8

Ebook: 978-1-968134-15-0

Printed in USA

ABOUT THE AUTHOR

As a certified trichologist and natural hair care educator, I specialize in helping individuals discover what's truly possible for their hair—especially when they've been told otherwise.

My passion lies in witnessing transformation—that moment when someone realizes their hair can be healthy, strong, and free. With a deep understanding of the science behind hair and scalp health, I strive to provide clarity, comfort, and actionable solutions. My training equips me to assess and guide care for a wide range of concerns, from common challenges like dandruff and dryness to complex conditions such as alopecia areata, scalp psoriasis, and CCCA.

But my work goes beyond diagnosis or technique. I believe in education, empowerment, and helping clients build routines that nourish their crown from root to tip. This includes learning to read labels, choosing products with purpose, avoiding harmful styling practices, and embracing care that fits their lifestyle and values.

While I offer expert insight from the field of trichology, I'm not a medical doctor. Hair and scalp symptoms can sometimes signal deeper health issues. That's why I encourage a holistic approach—and, when necessary, consulting licensed healthcare professionals for comprehensive support.

In this series, you'll find guidance rooted in science, experience, and care. My hope is that it not only helps you understand your hair better but also love it more, trust it more, and grow with it in ways you never thought possible.

Your hair is not the problem—you just needed the right guide.

DEDICATION

For the one craving consistency but lost in the chaos,
This is your rhythm. Your ritual.
Your return to ease.

OVERVIEW

Consistency is the key to thriving natural hair. *Build Your Routine* helps you create a care plan that works with your lifestyle—not against it. No more starting over every wash day or feeling overwhelmed by 10-step routines. This guide is about building habits you can actually stick to—and results you can actually see.

From daily moisture to monthly deep treatments, you'll map out a rhythm that supports healthy growth, strong strands, and stress-free maintenance.

SERIES INTRODUCTION

Welcome to *From Root to Tip: A Growing Hands Guide for Natural Hair*

This series was created with one goal in mind: to give you what's been missing—not just products, not just trends, but truth, support, and real guidance for real people who are ready to finally understand and care for their natural hair from the inside out.

For years, we've been taught to manage, fix, or fight our hair. But here, we're doing something different. We're returning to care—not control. To confidence. To consistency. To choice.

Each guide in this series is built as a step in your journey. They can be read in order or on their own, depending on where you are in your process. Whether you're just starting out, rebuilding your relationship with your hair, or deepening your understanding, this space is for you.

I've written these guides from my hands—growing hands that have touched, healed, protected, and restored countless crowns. Now, I offer that care to you.

This isn't just about hair. It's about healing. It's about reclaiming your rhythm, your confidence, and your beauty—from root to tip.

Let's begin.

WHAT YOU WILL LEARN

- How to break your regimen down into manageable steps
- The difference between maintenance, recovery, and treatment
- How to plan wash days that don't feel overwhelming
- When (and how) to trim, clarify, or adjust your routine
- How to adapt your care for seasons, hormones, or stress
- Tips for tracking growth, hydration, and overall hair health

WHAT YOU'LL WALK AWAY WITH

- A realistic, customized routine that honors your time and texture
- Tools to keep your regimen simple, effective, and consistent
- The flexibility to adapt your routine without guilt
- Peace of mind knowing you have a plan—and it works

TABLE OF CONTENTS

INTRODUCTION

There's no magic product—but there is a method. In *Build Your Routine*, we guide you through what a healthy natural hair routine really looks like. You'll learn how to organize your care into daily, weekly, and monthly tasks; how to listen to and adjust to your hair's changing needs; and how to track progress without pressure.

This isn't about perfection—it's about making your routine work for you. Whether you're a beginner or resetting after setbacks, this guide brings structure, clarity, and peace to your process.

Because when your routine is rooted in rhythm, your hair learns to trust you.

LESSON 1:
PERSONALIZED HAIR CARE PLANS

Developing a personalized hair care plan is essential for maintaining the health and beauty of natural textured hair. A well-structured routine addresses the specific needs of your hair type while seamlessly integrating into your lifestyle. This guide explores how to create a successful hair care regimen for Afro hair, focusing on tailoring the routine to individual needs and scheduling maintenance and treatments for optimal results.

Tailoring a Routine to Individual Hair Type and Lifestyle

1. Understanding Hair Types and Textures

The foundation of a personalized hair care plan begins with understanding your unique hair type and texture. Afro hair comes in a variety of textures, from loose curls to tight coils, each with its specific needs. Identifying whether your hair is type 4A, 4B, 4C, or a variation thereof helps in selecting the most effective products and techniques.

- **Type 4A:** Features a soft, S-shaped coil pattern with medium density, often prone to shrinkage. Moisturizing products that enhance curl definition and manage shrinkage work well for this type.

- **Type 4B:** Characterized by a zig-zag curl pattern that is less defined and often coarser. It requires heavy moisturizing and protective styling to minimize breakage.

- **Type 4C:** The most tightly coiled hair type, with minimal curl definition and a tendency toward dryness and shrinkage. This type benefits from routines focused on deep hydration and moisture retention.

2. Assessing Hair Needs and Goals

Understanding your hair type is only the beginning. Next, assess your hair's specific needs and goals. Are you looking to improve moisture levels, reduce breakage, or enhance curl definition? Evaluate your hair's current condition—dryness, brittleness, or split ends—to tailor your routine effectively.

3. Incorporating Lifestyle Factors

Your lifestyle plays a significant role in shaping your hair care routine. Consider the following:

- **Activity Level:** If you're frequently active or work out often, you might need a more frequent cleansing schedule to manage sweat and product buildup.

- **Climate:** Environmental conditions can influence hair health. For example, dry climates require additional moisturizing treatments, while humid climates may call for frizz control.

- **Time Commitment:** Your daily schedule determines how much time you can allocate to hair care. Creating a routine that fits your lifestyle ensures consistency and success.

4. Choosing the Right Products

Selecting the right products is key to addressing your hair's needs.

- **Shampoos and Conditioners:** Opt for sulfate-free shampoos to avoid stripping natural oils. Use conditioners that provide moisture and detangling benefits. Natural oils and butters, such as shea butter or jojoba oil, are especially beneficial.

- **Leave-In Conditioners and Moisturizers:** Lightweight but hydrating leave-ins maintain daily moisture.

- **Oils and Serums:** Oils like jojoba, argan, or olive oil help lock in moisture and add shine. Serums are excellent for managing frizz and protecting against environmental damage.

5. **Establishing a Routine**

A structured hair care routine is vital for maintaining healthy hair. Here's how to build a balanced regimen:

- **Cleansing:** Depending on your hair type and product usage, washing every two weeks may suffice. Over-washing can strip your hair of its natural oils, so adjust the frequency based on your scalp's needs.

- **Conditioning:** Deep conditioning should be a part of your routine at least once a month to restore moisture and strengthen your hair. Choose treatments tailored to your hair's specific needs, such as hydration, strengthening, or repair.

- **Moisturizing:** Regularly moisturizing—either daily or every other day—keeps hair hydrated. This can involve using leave-in conditioners, oils, or creams. For natural styles you prefer not to manipulate, moisturizing sprays work effectively without requiring frequent touch-ups.

Scheduling Maintenance and Treatments for Optimal Results

1. **Creating a Hair Care Calendar**

A hair care calendar helps you organize and track your routine. Include:

- **Cleansing and Conditioning:** Schedule specific days for washing and deep conditioning to maintain consistency.

- **Monthly Treatments:** Plan monthly moisture treatments to strengthen and hydrate your hair, enhancing retention and reducing breakage.

- **Quarterly Evaluations:** Every few months, assess your hair's health and adjust your routine as needed. This might involve switching products or techniques based on how your hair responds.

2. Implementing Protective Styles

Protective styles minimize manipulation and prevent breakage. Options like braids, twists, and updos shield your ends from damage. Schedule regular intervals for changing these styles to avoid strain on your hair and scalp.

3. Regular Trims

Trimming regularly helps remove split ends and maintain overall hair health. Depending on your hair's growth and condition, trims every 6–8 weeks prevent split ends from traveling up the hair shaft, reducing breakage and promoting healthier growth.

4. Monitoring Progress and Making Adjustments

Track how your hair responds to your routine. Observe changes in texture, moisture levels, and overall health. If you notice issues like increased breakage or dryness, reassess your routine.

Adjustments might include changing the frequency of washing, experimenting with different conditioning treatments, or refining your moisturizing techniques.

5. Integrating Healthy Habits

Beyond your hair care routine, incorporating healthy habits enhances your hair's overall condition:

- **Diet:** A balanced diet rich in vitamins and minerals supports hair health. Include nutrients like vitamin D, vitamin E, and omega-3 fatty acids.

- **Hydration:** Drinking plenty of water keeps your scalp hydrated from within.

- **Stress Management:** Managing stress through relaxation techniques or exercise can significantly impact hair health, as stress often causes excessive shedding.

By tailoring your hair care routine to your specific hair type, needs, and lifestyle, you can achieve optimal results. Maintaining a structured schedule for treatments and maintenance ensures your regimen aligns with your hair's unique requirements. A personalized approach leads to healthier, more vibrant natural hair while seamlessly fitting into your daily life.

LESSON 2:
WEEKLY AND MONTHLY MAINTENANCE

Maintaining the health and appearance of natural textured hair requires a structured approach to both weekly and monthly care. This guide focuses on creating a consistent routine for nourishment, upkeep, and preserving style and health between wash days.

Establishing a Routine for Regular Upkeep and Nourishment

1. Weekly Maintenance

Weekly maintenance is essential for keeping natural hair in optimal condition. This involves practices that cleanse, condition, and rejuvenate the hair.

- **Cleansing:** Washing your hair biweekly helps remove product buildup, excess oils, and impurities. Use a sulfate-free shampoo that gently cleanses without stripping essential moisture, focusing on the scalp where buildup typically accumulates. For those who find detangling during conditioning stressful, consider detangling during the shampoo process as follows:

  1. Wet hair thoroughly.

  2. Apply a light lather of shampoo with minimal manipulation.

  3. Detangle using the shampoo suds as a buffer to simplify the process.

- **Conditioning:** Apply a generous amount of conditioner from scalp to ends. Let it sit for 2–5 minutes to penetrate and hydrate the strands. Use a detangling brush to comb through for even distribution, then rinse thoroughly with cool water to seal in moisture.

- **Moisturizing:** After cleansing, your hair needs a moisturizing routine. Apply a leave-in conditioner and moisturizer to damp hair to lock in hydration and prepare it for styling. Opt for products containing humectants like glycerin or aloe vera, and seal the moisture in with oils or creams.

2. Monthly Maintenance

Monthly maintenance involves more intensive treatments and evaluations to ensure long-term hair health.

- **Scalp Treatments:** Address scalp concerns like dryness or dandruff with monthly treatments. Use scalp scrubs or oils infused with tea tree oil or peppermint to promote a healthy scalp environment, essential for optimal hair growth.

- **Deep Conditioning:** Deep conditioning treatments should be done monthly to restore moisture and strength. Choose a formula tailored to your hair's needs—hydrating, strengthening, or repairing. Apply generously from scalp to ends, and use a heat cap or steamer to enhance penetration. Allow the treatment to sit for the recommended time to fully nourish the hair.

- **Clarifying Treatments:** Use a clarifying shampoo to remove product buildup and hard water minerals. These shampoos offer a deeper clean than regular shampoos but should only be used occasionally, as they can strip natural oils. Follow with a moisturizing deep conditioner to restore hydration.

- **Protein Treatments:** Protein treatments strengthen hair by replenishing keratin. These treatments are particularly useful for hair prone to breakage or damaged by relaxers or coloring. However, ensure your hair is well-moisturized before applying protein treatments. Follow product instructions carefully, and always finish with a moisturizing deep conditioner to maintain a balance of protein and moisture.

3. Evaluating and Adjusting Your Routine

Remember, if it isn't broken, don't fix it. Many people get caught up in online videos showcasing various products and rush to buy whatever is trending. However, your hair deserves more thoughtful care than that. Products don't instantly fix issues, and just because you can feel a product on your hands doesn't mean your hair is moisturized.

The best way to determine if your hair is truly moisturized is to shampoo it and feel it after rinsing, with no products applied. If your hair feels squeaky, it's a sign that it's definitely dry.

At the end of each month, take time to evaluate your hair care routine. Look for signs such as changes in texture, moisture levels, and overall health. If you notice issues like increased breakage or dryness, adjust your routine accordingly. This may involve switching products, altering treatment frequency, or refining your techniques to better meet your hair's evolving needs

Techniques for Preserving Style and Health Between Wash Days

Keeping your hair healthy and maintaining your hairstyle between wash days requires strategic techniques to prevent damage and preserve its appearance.

1. Protecting Styles

Protective styles are essential for minimizing manipulation and preserving your hair's health. Styles like braids, twists, or updos help shield the ends of your hair and reduce exposure to environmental stressors. Be sure to install and remove these styles carefully to avoid tension or breakage.

- **Satin or Silk Scarves/Pillowcases:** Using satin or silk pillowcases or scarves reduces friction and moisture loss. These materials are much gentler on your hair compared to cotton, which can lead to dryness and breakage.

- **Loose Hairstyles:** If you prefer wearing your hair out, choose loose hairstyles that minimize tension on your scalp and hair shafts. Avoid tight styles that can cause breakage and scalp irritation.

2. Nighttime Care

A consistent nighttime routine is key to preserving both your hairstyle and hair health. Before bed, protect your hair using techniques such as:

- **Pineapple Method:** For curly or coily hair, loosely gather your hair at the top of your head and secure it with a silk or satin scarf. This helps maintain curl definition and prevents flattening or frizz.

- **Bantu Knots:** For stretched styles, bantu knots are an excellent option. They help maintain length and prevent tangling, making them ideal for transitioning between styles.

3. Mid-Week Refresh

Refreshing your hair between wash days can help maintain its appearance and manageability. Try these techniques:

- **Dry Shampoo:** For oily hair, apply a dry shampoo sparingly to absorb excess oil and refresh the scalp. Brush through to avoid product buildup.

- **Mist and Moisturize:** Lightly mist your hair with water or a moisturizing spray to rehydrate and redefine curls. Follow with a small amount of leave-in conditioner or oil to seal in moisture.

4. Avoiding Excessive Heat and Manipulation

Minimize the use of heat styling tools and excessive manipulation, as these can lead to damage and dryness. If heat styling is necessary, always use a heat protectant and opt for lower heat settings. Limit the frequency of heat styling to maintain your hair's health.

5. Regular Trims

Regular trims are vital for healthy hair. Trimming the ends every 6–8 weeks removes split ends and prevents breakage from traveling up the hair shaft. This practice promotes overall hair health and supports growth by keeping the ends in good condition.

By establishing a consistent weekly and monthly maintenance routine and incorporating strategies for preserving style and health between wash days, you can keep your natural textured hair vibrant, strong, and beautifully styled. Regular upkeep and thoughtful care not only enhance your hair's appearance but also support its long-term health and resilience.

LESSON 3:
TRACKING PROGRESS AND ADJUSTING ROUTINE

Monitoring Hair Growth and Overall Health

Monitoring your hair's progress and adapting your routine as needed are essential steps to maintaining healthy hair and promoting growth. This lesson outlines effective methods for tracking hair growth and overall health, as well as strategies for making adjustments based on your hair's changing needs.

Monitoring Hair Growth

1. Set Clear Goals

Start by setting clear and realistic goals to track your hair growth effectively. Determine how much length you want to achieve within a specific timeframe, such as three or six months.

Align these goals with your overall hair health aspirations. For example, if your primary goal is to increase length, focus on practices that support healthy growth, like regular trims and minimizing breakage.

2. Document Hair Length

Regularly measuring your hair length helps you monitor progress. Use a flexible measuring tape or ruler to measure from the root to the tip of your hair. Keep track of these measurements in a journal or a mobile app designed for tracking hair growth. Measure every 4–6 weeks to note gradual changes. Additionally, taking monthly photos provides a visual record of growth and highlights changes in texture and overall health.

3. Assess Hair Health

Hair health is about more than just length. Healthy hair should feel strong and resilient, exhibit natural shine, and be free of excessive breakage or split ends. Pay attention to key indicators like elasticity, moisture levels, and damage. Conduct a strand test to evaluate elasticity by gently stretching a strand of hair—healthy hair should stretch and return to its original length without snapping.

4. Monitor Scalp Condition

A healthy scalp is essential for optimal hair growth. Regularly check for signs of scalp issues, such as dryness, itching, or excessive oiliness. Maintaining a balanced scalp promotes a healthy environment for hair follicles. If you notice buildup or imbalances, consider using scalp treatments or exfoliants to restore scalp health.

Making Adjustments Based on Progress and Changing Needs

1. Adjusting Hair Care Products

As your hair grows and changes, so will its needs. Regularly assess and adjust the hair care products you use based on your current hair condition. For example, if you notice increased dryness, you might need to switch to more hydrating shampoos and conditioners. On the other hand, if your hair feels oily or weighed down, you may require lighter products or more frequent cleansing.

- **Hair Type and Texture:** Products that worked well in the past may no longer be effective as your hair grows or changes texture. For instance, you may need different styling products as your hair transitions from short to long. Regularly assess whether your products are still meeting your needs or if a change is necessary.

- **Scalp Health:** If your scalp's condition changes, adjust your routine accordingly. For example, if you develop a flaky scalp, consider using a medicated shampoo or scalp treatment. If your scalp becomes excessively oily, you may need a clarifying shampoo or a change in your moisturizing products.

2. Modify Routine Frequency

Based on your hair's progress and how it responds to your routine, you may need to adjust the frequency of certain practices. For example, if your hair becomes excessively dry, you might need to increase the frequency of deep conditioning treatments. On the other hand, if you notice signs of protein overload, reduce the frequency of protein treatments and focus more on moisturizing.

- **Washing Frequency:** Your hair type and scalp condition influence how often you should wash your hair. Some people may need to wash their hair more often to manage oil and build- up, while others benefit from less frequent washing to preserve natural oils. Adjust the frequency based on how your hair feels and looks.

- **Styling Practices:** If you notice excessive breakage or damage from certain styling practices, consider reducing their frequency or altering your techniques. For example, if frequent heat styling is causing damage, you might switch to heat-free styling methods or lower heat settings.

3. Incorporate Feedback and Observations

Pay attention to how your hair responds to different products and practices. Use feedback from your personal observations, as well as insights from others, to guide your routine. If a particular product or treatment works well, continue using it. However, if you notice negative effects or a lack of improvement, consider discontinuing or changing the product or method.

4. Adapt to Seasonal Changes

Seasonal shifts can affect your hair's needs. In winter, your hair may require additional moisture due to dry indoor air, while in summer, you might need products that protect against UV damage and chlorine. Adjust your routine to address the environmental factors that impact your hair health.

5. Seek Professional Advice

If you encounter persistent issues or are unsure how to adjust your routine, consider seeking advice from a hair care professional. A stylist or dermatologist can offer personalized recommendations based on your hair type, condition, and goals. They can also help diagnose underlying issues that may be affecting your hair's health.

6. Be Patient and Persistent

Hair growth and improvements in hair health take time. Be patient and persistent with your routine, and allow products and techniques time to show results. Regular monitoring and thoughtful adjustments will help you achieve and maintain healthy, vibrant hair.

By consistently monitoring your hair's progress and making informed adjustments to your routine, you can ensure that your hair remains healthy, strong, and beautiful. Adapting your hair care practices to meet your hair's evolving needs will support long-term success and help you achieve your hair goals.

QUIZ
CREATING A HAIR CARE ROUTINE

Lesson 1: Personalized Hair Care Plans

1. Question

What is the most important factor when creating a personalized hair care plan?

a) Using the most expensive products.

b) Tailoring the routine to your hair type and lifestyle.

c) Washing hair every day.

d) Following the same routine as someone with a different hair type.

Answer: b) Tailoring the routine to your hair type and lifestyle.

2. Question

Which of the following is crucial when scheduling maintenance and treatments for optimal hair health?

a) Only deep conditioning once a year.

b) Ignoring hair type and only focusing on scalp treatments.

c) Scheduling regular trims and deep conditioning based on hair needs.

d) Avoiding any oils or moisturizing treatments.

Answer: c) Scheduling regular trims and deep conditioning based on hair needs.

3. Question

Why is it important to tailor a hair care routine to an individual's lifestyle?

a) It helps minimize time spent on hair care.

b) It ensures the routine fits the person's daily habits and schedules for consistent results.

c) It allows more frequent salon visits.

d) It reduces the need for hair care altogether.

Answer: b) It ensures the routine fits the person's daily habits and schedules for consistent results.

Lesson 2: Weekly and Monthly Maintenance

1. Question

How often should weekly maintenance, such as conditioning and moisturizing, be performed?

a) Once a month.

b) Weekly, based on hair needs and type.

c) Daily for all hair types.

d) Never, unless hair is damaged.

Answer: b) Weekly, based on hair needs and type.

2. Question

Which of the following is a key technique for preserving hair style and health between wash days?

a) Reapplying heat to the hair daily.

b) Sleeping on a satin or silk pillowcase or using a satin bonnet.

c) Shampooing daily.

d) Avoiding moisturizing products.

Answer: b) Sleeping on a satin or silk pillowcase or using a satin bonnet.

3. Question

What should be included in a monthly hair care routine to ensure hair health?

a) A light oil treatment every day.

b) Deep conditioning treatments and scalp massages.

c) Frequent hair dyeing.

d) Applying heat styling tools regularly.

Answer: b) Deep conditioning treatments and scalp massages

4. **Question**

Which of the following is NOT recommended for weekly or monthly maintenance?

a) Trimming hair every two weeks.

b) Deep conditioning based on the moisture needs of the hair.

c) Using protective styles to reduce manipulation.

d) Hydrating hair with water-based moisturizers.

Answer: a) Trimming hair every two weeks.

Lesson 3: Tracking Progress and Adjusting Routine

1. Question

Why is it important to track hair growth over time?

a) To ensure hair grows evenly across the scalp.

b) To determine the effectiveness of the current hair care routine and make necessary adjustments.

c) To see how long the hair can grow without care.

d) To compare hair length with others.

Answer: b) To determine the effectiveness of the current hair care routine and make necessary adjustments.

2. Question

What is a good way to track your hair's progress over time?

a) Using heat styling tools to measure hair length.

b) Keeping a hair care journal with photos and notes about products and treatments.

c) Changing products monthly without measuring progress.

d) Not tracking at all and just observing growth casually.

Answer: b) Keeping a hair care journal with photos and notes about products and treatments.

3. Question

When should you adjust your hair care routine?

a) Only if you notice major hair breakage.

b) Every week, regardless of progress.

c) When you notice changes in your hair's needs or environment, such as weather or hair texture changes.

d) Never, once a routine is set.

Answer: c) When you notice changes in your hair's needs or environment, such as weather or hair texture changes.

CLOSING NOTE

Healthy hair doesn't come from hustle.
It comes from rhythm, rest, and routines that feel like
care—not chores.

www.ingramcontent.com/pod-product-compliance
Lightning Source LLC
Chambersburg PA
CBHW060615290326
41930CB00051B/2655